MEDICAL EXECUTIVE COMMITTEE

Essentials Handbook

Richard A. Sheff, MD

Robert J. Marder, MD

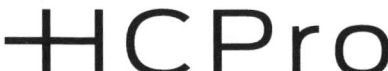

Medical Executive Committee Essentials Handbook is published by HCPro, Inc.

Copyright © 2012 HCPro, Inc.

All rights reserved. Printed in the United States of America.   5 4 3 2 1

ISBN: 978-1-60146-947-2

No part of this publication may be reproduced, in any form or by any means, without prior written consent of HCPro, Inc., or the Copyright Clearance Center (978-750-8400). Please notify us immediately if you have received an unauthorized copy.

HCPro, Inc., provides information resources for the healthcare industry.

HCPro, Inc., is not affiliated in any way with The Joint Commission, which owns the JCAHO and Joint Commission trademarks.

Richard A. Sheff, MD, Author
Robert J. Marder, MD, Author
Katrina Gravel, Editorial Assistant
Elizabeth Jones, Editor
Erin Callahan, Associate Editorial Director

Mike Mirabello, Graphic Artist
Matt Sharpe, Production Supervisor
Shane Katz, Art Director
Jean St. Pierre, Senior Director of Operations

Advice given is general. Readers should consult professional counsel for specific legal, ethical, or clinical questions.

Arrangements can be made for quantity discounts. For more information, contact:

HCPro, Inc.
75 Sylvan Street, Suite A-101
Danvers, MA 01923
Telephone: 800-650-6787 or 781-639-1872
Fax: 800-639-8511
Email: *customerservice@hcpro.com*

Visit HCPro online at: *www.hcpro.com* and *www.hcmarketplace.com*

Contents

Figure List vii

About the Authors ix

Chapter 1: Roles and Responsibilities of
the Medical Staff, Management, and Board 1

    Quality and Safety 1

    Board Responsibilities 4

    Medical Staff Responsibilities 8

    Management Responsibilities 9

    Understanding Influence 10

Chapter 2: The Power of the Pyramid: How to
Achieve Great Physician Performance 13

    Appoint Excellent Physicians 15

    Set, Communicate, and Achieve Buy-In to Expectations 16

    Measure Performance Against Expectations 20

    Provide Periodic Feedback 20

CONTENTS

    Manage Poor Performance 21

    Layers of the Performance Pyramid 24

Chapter 3: The MEC's Role in Credentialing and Privileging 33

    What Is Credentialing? 35

    What Is Privileging? 36

    Four Steps in the Credentialing and Privileging Process 37

    Policy in Action 41

    Essential Credentialing and Privileging Policies............................. 42

Chapter 4: The MEC's Role in Peer Review, Quality, and Patient Safety 45

    Assigning Roles and Responsibilities... 46

    Oversight of Ongoing and Focused Professional
    Practice Evaluations 49

    Managing Loose vs. Managing Tight 50

    Managing Systems Performance.. 51

    Patient Safety Basics.. 54

    Four Components of Patient Safety.. 56

    Organizational Performance Improvement..................................... 57

Chapter 5: The MEC's Role in Managing Professional Conduct 59

    Protecting a Culture of Safety 60

    Legal and Regulatory Obligation to Address Conduct Issues 60

CONTENTS

Create and Enforce Code of Conduct Policy 62

Performance Pyramid to Address Conduct 63

Chapter 6: The MEC's Role in Strategic Collaboration With the Hospital 67

The Right Number 68

The Right Type of Physician 69

The Right Quality 69

The Right Relationship to the Hospital 70

The Right Medical Staff Culture 71

The Right Structure and Processes 72

The Right Leadership 72

Chapter 7: Effective MEC Meetings 75

Developing the MEC Agenda 75

MEC Members' Role in Meeting Effectiveness 78

Figure List

Figure 1.1 Organizational chart 6

Figure 1.2 Three legged stool 7

Figure 1.3 Sphere of control, influence, interest 12

Figure 2.1 The bad apple theory vs. performance improvement 14

Figure 2.2 The physician performance pyramid 15

Figure 2.3 Comparison of The Joint Commission's General Physician Competencies with the Physician Performance Pyramid dimensions 19

Figure 2.4 ACPE/Greeley dimensions of physician performance 26

Figure 2.5 ACGME/The Joint Commission dimensions of physician performance 27

FIGURE LIST

Figure 3.1 The medical staff's major functions 33

Figure 4.1 What is practitioner performance? 47

Figure 4.2 Why do events happen? 55

About the Authors

Richard A. Sheff, MD

Richard A. Sheff, MD, is principal and chief medical officer with The Greeley Company, a division of HCPro, Inc., in Danvers, Mass. He brings more than 25 years of healthcare management and leadership experience to his work with physicians, hospitals, and healthcare systems across the country. With his distinctive combination of medical, healthcare, and management acumen, Dr. Sheff develops tailored solutions to the unique needs of physicians and hospitals. He consults, authors, and presents on a wide range of healthcare management and leadership issues, including governance, physician-hospital alignment, medical staff leadership development, emergency department call, peer review, hospital performance improvement, disruptive physician management, conflict resolution, physician employment and contracting, healthcare systems, service line management, hospitalist program optimization, patient safety and error reduction, credentialing, strategic planning, regulatory compliance, and helping physicians rediscover the joy of medicine.

Robert J. Marder, MD

Robert J. Marder, MD, is an advisory consultant and director of medical staff services with The Greeley Company, a division of HCPro, Inc., in Danvers, Mass. He brings more than 25 years of healthcare leadership and management experience to his work with physicians, hospitals, and healthcare organizations across the country. Dr. Marder's many roles in senior hospital medical administration and operations management in academic and community hospital settings make him uniquely qualified to assist physicians and hospitals in developing solutions for complex medical staff and hospital performance issues. He consults, authors, and presents on a wide range of healthcare leadership issues, including effective and efficient peer review, physician performance measurement and improvement, hospital quality measurement systems and performance improvement, patient safety/error reduction, and utilization management.

DOWNLOAD YOUR MATERIALS NOW

This handbook includes a customizable presentation that organizations can use to train physician leaders. The presentation complements the information provided in this handbook and can be downloaded at the following link:

www.hcpro.com/downloads/10554

Thank you for purchasing this product!

HCPro

CHAPTER 1

Roles and Responsibilities of the Medical Staff, Management, and Board

Many times physicians find themselves in leadership positions without the training needed to understand and carry out the responsibilities of the position. All too often, the medical executive committee (MEC) is comprised of a group of physicians who, though willing to contribute to the committee's goals, lack the knowledge and skill necessary to do so most effectively. Leadership training is not part of most medical school curricula or residency training.

In this chapter, we will address the roles and responsibilities of the medical staff, management, and the board. Think about these roles within the context of "good fences make good neighbors." A hospital cannot run effectively unless leaders understand and respect the roles each of these groups play.

Quality and Safety

The answer to the question, "Who is responsible for the quality and safety of care at the hospital?" can vary depending on who you

CHAPTER 1

ask. Some might say that physicians hold this responsibility. Physicians care for patients, write the orders, determine courses of care, and are often the ones sued if anything goes wrong. Another person may answer that the entire medical staff is responsible for quality of care and still another might assert that the hospital management is responsible. The trouble is that if everyone is responsible, it is difficult to hold someone accountable. The buck has to stop somewhere.

At the hospital, the buck stops with the governing board. However, that doesn't mean physicians and hospital management are off the hook. Anyone who interacts with the patient or touches anything that ultimately touches the patient is responsible for his or her role in patient care. Every individual is responsible for his or her own actions. But, at the end of the day, ultimate responsibility for quality of care rests with the board.

The governing board's responsibility for quality of care is tied to the concept of corporate negligence. The theory behind corporate negligence is that if a person or organization violates an assigned duty and that violation results in injury or harm, the person or organization is liable for that harm. When corporate negligence cases were first brought to the courts, the subjects of such cases were typically railroad and steel companies. Hospitals were off limits because they were seen as charitable organizations and therefore could not be sued under the principle of charitable immunity. That all changed in 1965 in a legal case in Illinois known as *Darling vs. Charleston Memorial Hospital*. In that case, a young

ROLES AND RESPONSIBILITIES OF THE MEDICAL STAFF

man came to the emergency room with a broken leg. The physician who set the leg did not have a lot of experience doing so. The young man was eventually admitted to the hospital suffering from gangrene and ultimately lost his foot to an amputation. His family sued the physician and the hospital. One of the charges against the hospital was that it granted the physician privileges for a procedure for which he was not competent to perform. The court found in the patient's favor. This was the first time that corporate negligence was applied to hospitals.

There have since been many court decisions that make clear that the governing board is responsible for the quality of care in the hospital. Does this precedent mean that if a physician removes a patient's right foot instead of the left that the board is responsible? If a dangerous dose of medication is administered because the physician misplaced the decimal point, is the board responsible for the resulting harm? The answer to both these questions is "yes." With that said, the physician has a duty to perform his or her duties well. The medical staff has a duty to conduct credentialing, privileging, and peer review. But all these responsibilities roll up to the governing board, which begs the question, "What does the board know about quality and safety of medical care?" The most common answer is not a lot. That's a problem and that's where the organized medical staff comes into play.

Quality standards adopted by the American College of Surgeons in the early 1900s established that hospitals must have an organized medical staff with healthcare expertise and that is responsible for quality of medical care. Since the inception of the organized medical staff, governing boards have delegated responsibilities for monitoring and improving the quality of care to the medical staff and to management. This delegation of responsibilities complicates matters as many medical staffs and management struggle to determine who was responsible for what.

Board Responsibilities

Distilled down to the basics, the board's primary responsibilities are to preserve and enhance the financial assets of the organization and to achieve high-quality care for patients. The board is challenged to balance "dollars" and quality—not one at the expense of the other. Many times physicians assert, "Quality trumps cost." Management then pushes back and says, "No money, no mission." The truth is that they're both right. At a time when the cost for care often exceeds the reimbursement for that care, the organization must balance quality of patient care with the cost-effectiveness of care.

Boards also establish the organization's mission, vision, values, and the strategic plan. The board also adopts financial targets and quality targets. Developing a budget and financial targets is the easier task of the two. While generally accepted accounting principles are well established, the board has few guidelines to follow when developing quality targets. The board also has the authority to grant medical staff membership and privileges. The medical staff makes recommendations concerning membership and privileges to the board, but it is the governing board that makes the final decision.

Boards are the ultimate conflict-resolving entity in the organization. When a conflict percolates up to the board, it owns the discussion and ultimate decision whether the issue is related to peer review, a turf battle, or physician-hospital conflict that can't be resolved. Keep in mind that the board carries out many of its responsibilities by delegating tasks and ensuring accountability. For example, the board delegates to management the responsibility to achieve financial targets and holding management accountable through periodic reviews of financial reports. Similarly, the board delegates responsibility for physician performance to the medical staff and holds the medical staff accountable for carrying out those responsibilities.

The board is also responsible for compliance legal and regulatory requirements and for ensuring patient, worker, and visitor safety.

That's a lot of responsibility, which is why it is important to acknowledge the difference between management and governance. Governance is a 30,000-foot view of responsibility. As noted earlier, boards are the ultimate conflict-resolving entity. They must rely on others within the organization. For example, the board must recruit and hire an effective CEO, set clear performance expectations for him or her to meet, and continually measure his

CHAPTER 1

or her performance and provide feedback. The board must also ensure that the CEO has adequate resources to fulfill his or her responsibilities.

Organizational chart

To understand the MEC's role, you must first understand the relationship among other groups on the organizational chart (see Figure 1.1). The governing board hires the CEO, who hires the vice presidents, who then hire the directors, etc. The board delegates these hiring decisions to the CEO, who then delegates to the management team. The board holds the management team accountable by holding the CEO accountable.

By drilling down on the organizational chart a bit more, it becomes clear that the MEC makes recommendations to the governing board regarding credentialing and privileging decisions. The general medical staff reserves the power to amend bylaws and elect officers. The medical staff can also report/recommend directly to

Figure 1.1

ORGANIZATIONAL CHART

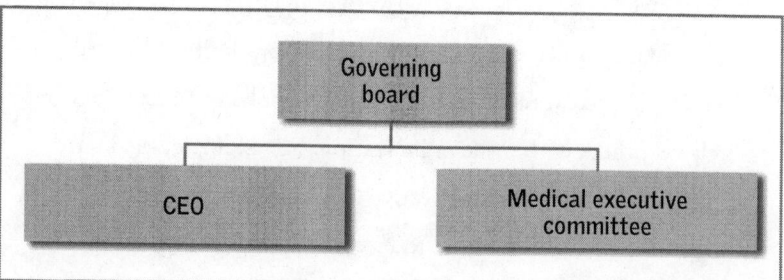

ROLES AND RESPONSIBILITIES OF THE MEDICAL STAFF

the board if it determines the need to override the MEC, but such events should be few and far between.

The organizational chart described here is the most common at hospitals today. However, there is another organizational chart that's alive and kicking. This "three-legged stool" approach arises when the medical staff throws up a red flag and says, "We are not subservient to the board. We should be an equal partner, an equal voice to management to the board and in some cases stand over and against the board and management." In some ways, the three-legged stool model is an advocacy model (see Figure 1.2).

When the medical staff is advocating for patient care quality, it is carrying out its board-delegated responsibility for quality of care for which it is held accountable. But when the medical staff is advocating for physicians, it is following the three-legged stool model. In this case, the medical staff wants to be seen and engaged as a partner with management and the board to accomplish physician success, hospital success, and good-quality patient care.

Figure 1.2   THREE LEGGED STOOL

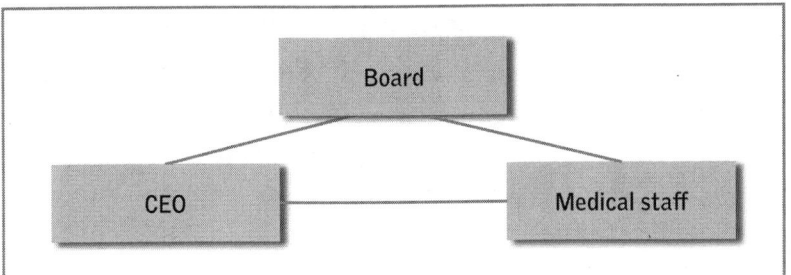

The three-legged stool approach is a way of ensuring that the organization is not overvaluing one of those at the expense of any others.

The take-home message is that the organization is structured to hold physicians accountable to the board in a hierarchical relationship and, at the same time, to encourage physicians to partner with the board and hospital to achieve shared objectives. Keep these two organizational charts in mind and understand that both models are often at play.

Medical Staff Responsibilities

The board delegates to the medical staff the responsibility for monitoring and improving the quality of care that is primarily dependent on the performance of individuals granted privileges. For example, a patient comes to the emergency room complaining of abdominal pain. The surgeon diagnoses cholecystitis, performs good preop stabilization, takes the patient to the operating room, demonstrates strong technique, provides good postop care, and achieves a great clinical outcome. The medical staff owns the surgeon's actions that resulted in the good clinical outcome. However, the clinical outcome is also dependent on the competence of nurses, lab techs, etc. The medical staff does not "own" these other parts of the process.

ROLES AND RESPONSIBILITIES OF THE MEDICAL STAFF

To monitor and improve quality of care, the medical staff has organized itself into a self-governed structure. The model of self-governance presents challenges as healthcare becomes more and more complicated. Balancing costs, physician-hospital competition, financial dependence/referral relationships, and patient safety challenges make self-governance difficult. Again, the medical staff is assigned responsibility for the quality of care delivered by the medical staff, which means that physicians are mutually accountable to each other.

Management Responsibilities

Management is also responsible for meeting board-approved quality and financial performance targets and for ensuring compliance with regulatory requirements. Management must also ensure that the organization has adequate staff and facilities to meet these targets.

Management also provides resources to the board and the medical staff to help these groups fulfill their responsibilities. For example, the medical staff services department aids the medical staff by providing credentialing and regulatory expertise, and the quality management department partners with the medical staff to ensure effective peer review.

Physician executives or medical directors, vice presidents of medical affairs (VPMA), or chief medical officers (CMO) may also guide the medical staff. These physician executives fall under the CEO on the organizational chart. They are hired by, are compensated by, and are accountable to the CEO. The physician executives are not directly accountable to the medical staff, and the medical staff is not directly accountable to them. However, they are often a resource for and have influence on the medical staff.

Understanding Influence

What happens if a medical staff doesn't fulfill its responsibilities? Often, the CEO, VPMA, or CMO get pulled into the space between the board and the MEC to intervene. However, doing so usurps the role of the medical staff. Medical staffs must remember that if it fails to self-govern, to hold one another mutually accountable through effective quality, patient safety, peer review, and credentialing policies, the power will be taken out of its hands. The board has the authority to make that decision.

We return again to the idea of good fences making good neighbors. The medical staff owns physician performance issues. Physicians care about everything that happens to the patient—from admitting the patient, to treating the patient, to delivering meals. All these things fall within the physician's sphere of influence. Unfortunately, not all these things fall within the physician's sphere of control.

ROLES AND RESPONSIBILITIES OF THE MEDICAL STAFF

But things that fall into the medial staff's sphere of influence are critical to hospital operations. The medical staff can influence important decisions, such as staffing and strategic planning. In line with Joint Commission standards, the department chair has input into staffing within his or her department. The medical staff can also have an influence over the hospital's strategic planning, which is owned by the board. Further, the physician can influence the other practitioner's actions. For example, the physician can educate the nurse about the patient's condition and share the treatment plan with the nurse. The physician can also make clear that he or she is worried about the patient's condition and encourage the nurse to call should the patient's condition change overnight. Doing so expands the physician's sphere of influence.

As illustrated in Figure 1.3, the medical staff has a sphere of control, a sphere of influence, and a sphere of interest. As you can see, the sphere of control is much smaller than the sphere of influence and sphere of interest. The organized medical staff has an interest in everything that goes on at the hospital. The medical staff is interested in patient care, the hospital's reputation and financial standing, the physician plant, and the competence of all staff. But, again, the medical staff's sphere of control is limited to those tasks delegated to them by the board—the quality of care primarily dependent upon performance of individuals granted privileges.

Figure 1.3

SPHERE OF CONTROL, INFLUENCE, INTEREST

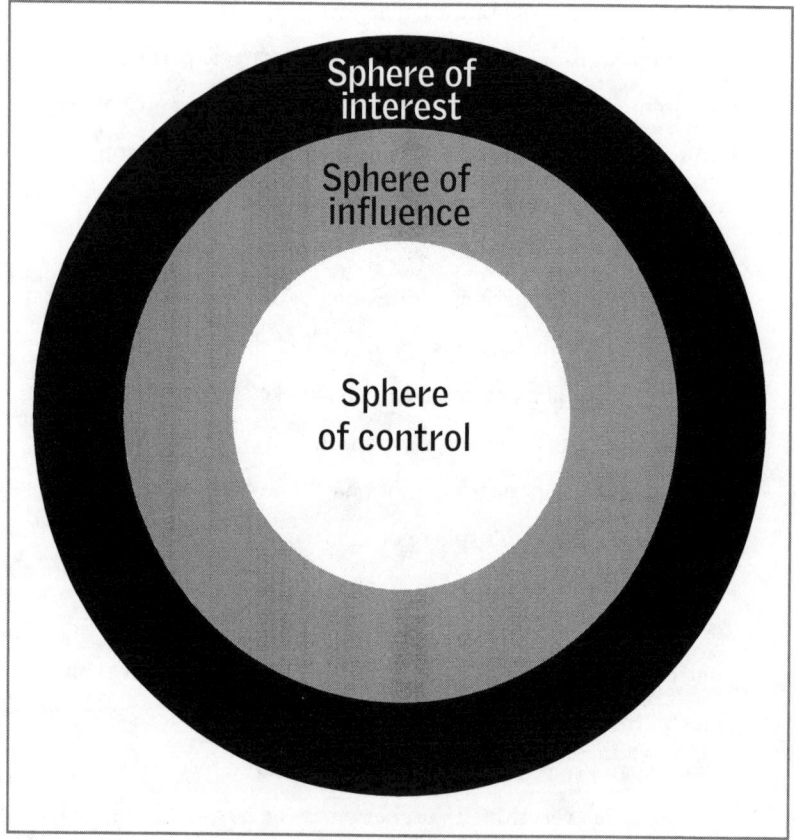

When keeping in mind these three spheres, it's important to recognize that the better the medical staff addresses the issues within its sphere of control, the better it can address things that fall within the spheres of influence and interest and expand the medical staff's ability to help the hospital and fellow physicians achieve mutual goals.

CHAPTER 2

The Power of the Pyramid: How to Achieve Great Physician Performance

As discussed in Chapter 1, the primary role of the MEC is to improve the performance of all members of the medical staff. To do that well, many hospitals have adopted the "Power of the Pyramid," which is an HR model introduced by the American College of Physician Executives. The Power of the Pyramid aims to achieve great physician performance by reducing conflict and increasing efficiency toward helping every physician to be the best that he or she can be.

The traditional model of performance improvement followed a "bad apples" approach. The organization would find negative outliers and ask him or her to "do better." The problem with using this bell-shaped curve, as illustrated in Figure 2.1 below, was that new "negative outliers" constantly emerged as some physicians improved performance—there was never improvement to the overall performance of the organization.

Figure 2.1

THE BAD APPLE THEORY VS. PERFORMANCE IMPROVEMENT

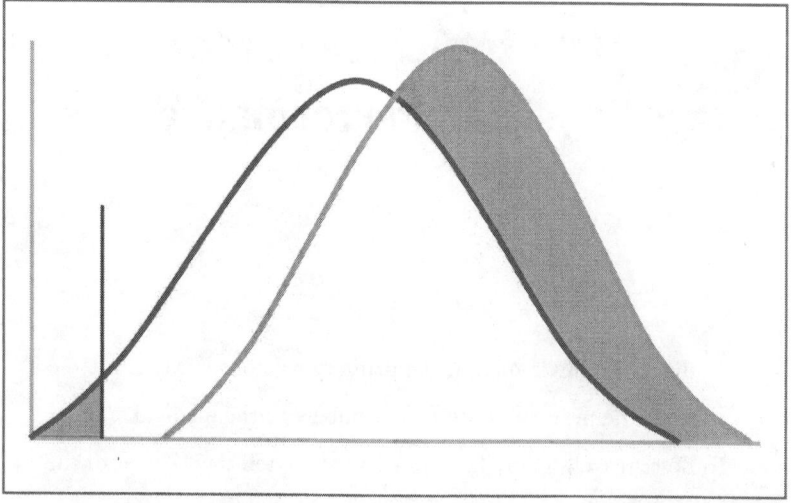

The organization should focus not just on improving individual performance but also on improving the performance of the entire medical staff—whether the individual physician falls on the lower, middle, or upper end of the curve. This approach moves away from the punitive culture bred by the "bad apple" theory and creates a positive culture of performance improvement.

When following the Power of the Pyramid, the goal is to spend the most time on the foundation layers to minimize the amount of time spent on the top layer of the pyramid—corrective action. Figure 2.2 depicts the physician performance pyramid.

THE POWER OF THE PYRAMID

Figure 2.2

The Physician Performance Pyramid

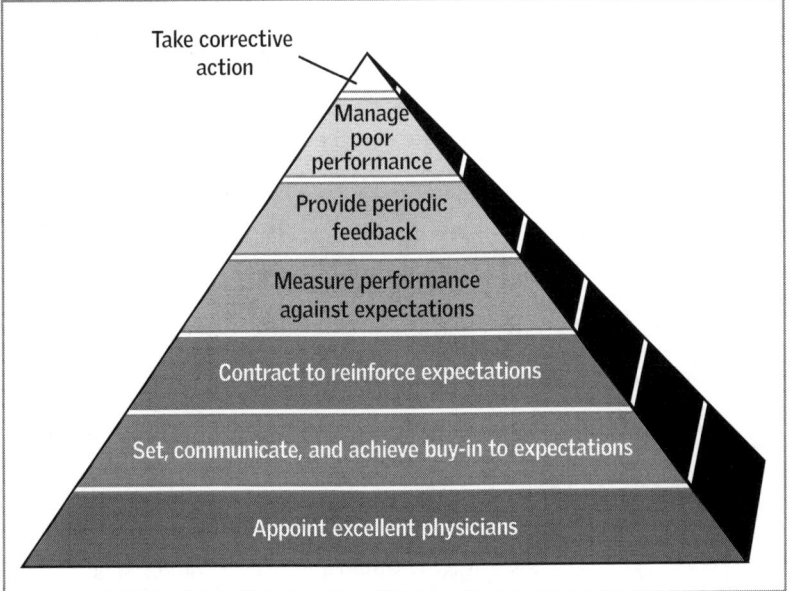

Appoint Excellent Physicians

Strong physician performance begins with credentialing and privileging. The very best way to address any performance issue is at the door, either at appointment or reappointment. Department chairs should sit down with applicants and go through the expectations of them as medical staff members and as members of the clinical department. At reappointment, department chairs should meet with problematic practitioners who are struggling with performance issues and review performance expectations and gauge their willingness to commit to meeting those expectations.

The best possible time to review expectations and discuss performance is at appointment and reappointment. Once the physician gets in the door, or the door is reopened to the physician, the problem is for the department chair to manage for up to the next two years. To be as proactive as possible, department chairs should address performance issues at this layer of the pyramid. Use the organization's eligibility criteria for both membership and privileges as a guide. Because the department chair recommends eligibility criteria to the credentials committee, the MEC, and the governing board, it's critically important that he or she sets the bar at a level that he or she feels comfortable implementing and enforcing. Remember that when the department chair helps to address the policies and procedures around credentialing and privileging, he or she must consider the behavioral issues that should be addressed at this layer of the pyramid.

Set, Communicate, and Achieve Buy-In to Expectations

The next layer of the pyramid is critically important, and one that medical staffs don't always do well—setting, communicating, and achieving buy-in to expectations. Department chairs should strive to articulate written expectations when interviewing an applicant at appointment, at reappointment, and when performance issues arise. For example, if the department chair has a team member who struggles with medical records, the chair is better able to address and resolve that issue if he or she has clearly articulated expectations about performing medical records and has explained the impact of incomplete medical records on the institution financially and on patient safety. Put these expectations in writing, have department members sign off, and address any concerns, differences of opinion, or lack of buy-in at that point.

Don't forget that performance expectations go beyond technical expectations to include multiple performance dimensions. Create a framework in which to define what it means to be a good physician practitioner in your clinical department and on the medical staff.

If you recall, these are the American College of Physician Executives (ACPE) and Greeley expectations:

- Technical quality of care

- Quality of service

- Patient safety/patient rights

- Resource utilization

- Peer and coworker relationships

- Citizenship

Or, you might choose the ACGME and the Joint Commission dimensions of physician performance, which include:

- Patient care

- Medical/clinical knowledge

- Practice-based learning and improvement

- Interpersonal and communication skills

- Professionalism

- Systems-based practice

There is a great deal of overlap between the ACPE and the ACGME performance expectations, as shown in Figure 2.3.

It is essential that you choose a framework with which to define what it means to be a good practitioner in your clinical department and on the medical staff. Department chairs should accept responsibility for recommending a framework to the quality committee and the credentials committee. These committees will then recommend a framework to the MEC and the governing board.

Figure 2.3 **COMPARISON OF THE JOINT COMMISSION'S GENERAL PHYSICIAN COMPETENCIES WITH THE PHYSICIAN PERFORMANCE PYRAMID DIMENSIONS**

Joint Commission / Pyramid	Patient Care	Medical Knowledge	Practice Based Learning	Interpersonal/Communication Skills	Professionalism	Systems Based Practices
Technical Quality	X	X	X			
Service Quality	X			X		X
Patient Safety/Rights	X		X		X	X
Resource Use	X	X	X			X
Relationships				X	X	
Citizenship					X	X

Measure Performance Against Expectations

Once you set, articulate, and achieve buy-in to expectations, you want to measure performance against expectations. Department chairs should recommend to the quality committee performance metrics with two targets: one to recognize excellence, and the other to recognize good performance and to separate good performance from performance that needs follow-up. This will be part of a practitioner's feedback report or ongoing professional practice evaluation, which is part of the department chair's responsibilities. We'll talk more about this role later in this training handbook. The key point to remember is that the department chair should set performance benchmarks and metrics in which to assess and measure and improve physician performance.

Provide Periodic Feedback

The quality committee, with oversight from the MEC, should provide a feedback report to physicians every six to eight months. The department chair should review these reports with individual practitioners in the department. Providing physicians with these reports, and engaging them in a discussion about the data, provides practitioners with the opportunity to correct their clinical performance.

Department chairs should be prepared for physicians to push back on the data and say the data are imperfect. Remind physicians that they are in a profession that is both art and science. Although it's easy to measure objective data for a science, it's extremely problematic to measure performance data for an art. If physicians fail to buy in to expectations or if they can't measure up to your performance expectations through metrics or if they won't respond constructively to feedback, you need to move to the next level of the pyramid to manage poor performance.

Manage Poor Performance

Managing poor performance is a pyramid within a pyramid, comprised of the following four layers:

1. **Collegial intervention.** The first layer is collegial intervention. If an issue arises—whether it's related to conduct, noncompliance with core measures, or noncompliance with the medical records policy—the department chair should first engage in a collegial dialogue with the practitioner and help him or her understand why this is an important performance measure or expectation. Help the physician understand why it's an important component of overall performance assessment. Ideally, get the physician to document his or her willingness to comply and/or work with the department chair toward improvement. The department

chair should also sign that document. If the physician fails to improve his or her performance following this discussion, the organization must move to the next step of creating a voluntary action plan.

2. **Voluntary action plan.** A physician may balk at creating an action plan, in which case the department chair must tell him or her, "If you're unwilling to create and follow a voluntary action plan, we'll have to develop a mandatory action plan, and that is far less collegial." Typically, most physicians will want to maintain as much autonomy and freedom as possible and will opt for the voluntary action plan. Within a voluntary action plan, address improvement that is measurable and include both positive and negative consequences for compliance with the plan. Also include time frames. For example, make it clear that if the physician complies with the voluntary improvement plan within three months, the organization will go back to purely collegial intervention.

3. **Mandatory action plan.** If the voluntary action plan is unsuccessful, the next layer of the pyramid is a mandatory action plan. The department chair should draft this improvement plan with oversight of the MEC and the quality committee. Ensure that the action plan includes measurable data (for example, requiring that the physician cut medical record deficiencies or validated complaints in half).

THE POWER OF THE PYRAMID

Have the physician sign the plan, sign it yourself, and create a time frame for compliance. For example, consider including a statement that says that if the physician complies with the mandatory improvement plan for six to 12 months, he or she will then move to a voluntary improvement plan for three months, and if able to successfully comply with that for three months, he or she will move down the pyramid to purely collegial intervention.

4. **Final warning.** Finally, the upper part of this part of the pyramid is what we call the "doc in the box" letter or final warning. At this stage, the organization (department chair, MEC, and governing board) must state exactly what the physician must do to avoid corrective action. Document opportunities for improvement and specific performance metrics and time frames. Again, consider including positive consequences even in a final warning, stating that if the physician complies with the parameters set out in the final warning, he or she can go back to a mandatory action plan, back to a voluntary action plan, and back to purely collegial intervention.

5. **Take corrective action.** Should the final warning fail to result in performance improvement, the organization must move into corrective action. Corrective action is any step the organization takes that decreases a physician's current clinical privileges or political membership rights on the medical

staff. Again, the organization should want to do everything possible to focus on the foundation layers of the pyramid, taking preventive and proactive actions, to avoid having to take corrective action. Understand that if you absolutely must "splash the cold water in someone's face" because they won't or can't take steps to improve performance, you can issue a precautionary suspension for up to 14 days without having to offer due process rights and up to 30 days without having to make a report to the National Practitioner Data Bank.

Note: An additional step is added to the performance pyramid when it comes to contracted members of the medical staff in your clinical department. Service agreements and professionals or exclusive contracts should include performance metrics, targets, and positive and negative consequences of complying with these expectations. Should a performance issue arise, not only does the department chair, the MEC, and the governing board have authority, but whomever signs their contract also has legally binding authority to hold the physician accountable.

Layers of the Performance Pyramid

The base of the pyramid is credentialing and privileging, because the best predictor of future performance is past performance. Initial appointment and reappointment is the best opportunity to address performance issues. The way to do this is by setting well-researched credentialing and privileging criteria—criteria for membership and criteria for exercising requested privileges. Once a physician is granted membership and privileges, his or her performance is a concern of the MEC for the next two years. It's important at reappointment to assess the data gathered through ongoing professional practice evaluation (OPPE) to determine physician competence. Should performance data indicate a need for improvement, take immediate steps to partner with the physician to help him or her improve.

The next layer of the pyramid is setting, communicating, and achieving physician buy-in to expectations. Hospitals frequently struggle with this layer of the pyramid that requires the organization to establish a framework for performance, set and establish communication and performance expectations, and set expectations for physicians in regard to service, patient safety, patient rights, interpersonal conduct, and citizenship. After setting these expectations, the organization must get the physicians' buy-in. For example, a physician who consistently fails to complete medical records likely never bought into the importance of completing medical records. Further, a physician who is consistently labeled as "disruptive" was likely not trained that conduct has value in terms of performance and standing on the medical staff.

To set and communicate expectations, consider adopting the example performance frameworks depicted in Figure 2.4 below. These frameworks, developed by the ACPE and The Greeley Company, include technical quality of care, quality of service, patient safety, patient rights, resource utilization, peer and coworker relationships, and citizenship. In addition, the ACGME and The Joint Commission created general competencies that address patient care, medical clinical knowledge, practice-based learning and improvement, interpersonal communication skills, professionalism, and systems-based practice. As shown in Figure 2.5, there is overlap between the ACGME and Joint Commission competencies. Whether you are a Joint Commission–accredited hospital or not, it is important that you adopt a framework of performance through which you can define what it means to be a good practitioner on your medical staff.

The third layer of the pyramid is measuring performance against expectations. That means taking performance indicators with

Figure 2.4 **ACPE/GREELEY DIMENSIONS OF PHYSICIAN PERFORMANCE**

• Technical quality of care
• Quality of service
• Patient safety/patient rights
• Resource utilization
• Peer and coworker relationships
• Citizenship

Figure 2.5

ACGME/The Joint Commission dimensions of physician performance

- Patient care
- Medical/clinical knowledge
- Practice-based learning and improvement
- Interpersonal and communication skills
- Professionalism
- Systems-based practice

benchmarks or targets, and we recommend having two targets to recognize excellence and establish indicators within each performance dimension. Communicate that to members of the medical staff, and then that can be made up to create the framework of your OPPE. Then every six to eight months, provide feedback to physicians on the medical staff in the form of a feedback report. Also, provide feedback reports to anyone granted clinical privileges, which may include physicians, podiatrists, psychologists, maxillofacial surgeons, and allied health professionals who are granted privileges. These individuals we now call advanced practice professionals. And the best part of providing provider feedback is that it enables each practitioner to manage their own clinical practice and to achieve improvements on their own without any intervention from leadership.

The next layer of the pyramid is the most challenging. It is how to manage poor or marginal performance, and this is a pyramid within a pyramid. You may have department chairs who feel comfortable implementing this layer of the pyramid, and you may have department chairs who don't feel comfortable doing this. But typically it starts with a collegial dialogue. Have a dialogue with your colleagues where you sit down, go over the performance issue, frame it in measurable terms, and give them the opportunity to improve.

How do we do this? Typically, a best practice is creating a letter of agreement where you state the issue, you have them sign it, agreeing to work with you on this issue, and then you sign it as a medical leader. This will require that you as a leader offer support or resources to them to do it. If that doesn't work, you may go onto the next step of managing poor performance, which is creating a voluntary action plan. If the practitioner is not interested in doing this, you may have to say, "If you're unable to do a voluntary action plan, we may ask you to do a mandatory action plan, which is not in your interest." State in the voluntary action plan that if the physician is successful in compliance with that over a three- to six-month period, whatever you decide is your time frame, then you can go back to a purely collegial interaction.

The next layer of the pyramid is a mandatory improvement action, and typically this would be something measurable. For example, if it's a medical record violation, you may say, "We'd like you to cut your violations in half," or if it's a conduct issue, "We'd like you to cut the number of validated complaints in half over a six- to

12-month period. If you're able to do that, then we'll go back to a purely collegial relationship or a voluntary action plan."

"Doc in the box," or the final warning, is where the person is told he or she must modify his or her conduct. He or she must modify his or her medical records or whatever the performance issue is, and this is what will happen if he or she doesn't. State how you will know if he or she doesn't do it and the consequences of not doing it.

Finally, taking corrective action under the Health Care Quality Improvement Act would limit his or her privileges or membership rights as a member of the organized medical staff.

Looking at the whole pyramid together, you can see that you should focus on the foundation layers of the pyramid. You want to address issues at appointment and reappointment. You want to create a quality framework and, most importantly, have the critical dialogues with practitioners so that you can obtain their buy-in. The bias of Dr. Howard Kerrs was that if you don't have their buy-in, you need to keep meeting until you get the buy-in, because there's no point attempting to measure performance if you don't have their understanding and insight as to what the criticality of this performance issue is. Then you want to meet with the quality committee to create performance measures and benchmarks, and having two targets is recommended: one target to recognize excellence, and the other target to separate good performance from adequate performance or performance that needs further information or follow-up.

At the next layer of the pyramid, you want to create your performance feedback reports, and then and only then, if you have a performance issue, should you manage poor performance. They might ask how taking corrective action is still helping a physician to be the best that he or she can be.

Imagine a scenario in which you have been working with a colleague for years regarding his alcoholism, giving him multiple warnings and multiple opportunities to go to rehab. Finally, he comes into the intensive care unit intoxicated and you are forced to intervene and take over patient care after hours. Following the incident, you would need to sit down with this physician and explain why you needed to summarily suspend him from the medical staff. You could give him the opportunity to take a medical leave of absence to go through rehab and hopefully come back sober in the future. The physician may be furious when you first take the corrective action, but with time he may realize that you are supporting him in the best way possible and helping him make necessary changes to his life. And that's the key with the performance pyramid.

Increasingly, physicians are either employed today or contracted by healthcare organizations. This provides an opportunity for another layer of the pyramid. So after you set, communicate, and achieve buy-in to expectations, you actually want to contract to reinforce those expectations. This is a new layer of the pyramid, and it's an opportunity for you to put the expectations, the performance measures, and the targets directly into the contracts. Now employed physicians will have a dual accountability, where they're accountable to the MEC for the overall performance and conduct and also accountable to their employer for the terms of the contract.

As you'll see from looking at the final layer of the pyramid, you want to focus on the opportunities to help to improve performance, establish performance of credentialing and privileging, measure performance, provide feedback, and then and only then manage poor performance and take corrective action.

Hopefully you'll be able to use this model that Howard Kerrs crafted so well and help physicians to improve and prevent having to do anything that would be perceived as disciplinary or negative or something contrary to what you're trying to establish to create a collegial culture.

CHAPTER 3

The MEC's Role in Credentialing and Privileging

In this chapter, we'll discuss the MEC's role in credentialing and privileging in more detail. As discussed in Chapter 1, credentialing and privileging are two of the primary functions delegated to the medical staff by the governing board. To understand the MEC's role in credentialing and privileging, we must first look at how these functions fit in with the organized structure of the medical staff. Again, we reference the organizational chart to illustrate the MEC's role (see Figure 3.1).

Figure 3.1   THE MEDICAL STAFF'S MAJOR FUNCTIONS

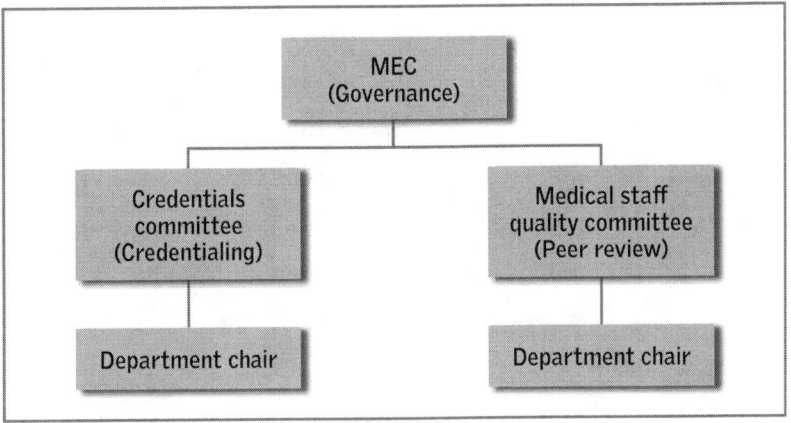

The MEC has overall governance responsibility for the medical staff. There are some reserved responsibilities of the general medical staff, which include election of officers, bylaws development and amendments, and the ability to go around the MEC and directly to the board in some instances. However, the MEC oversees all medical staff self-governance activities—including credentialing and privileging.

At most hospitals, the credentials committee is responsible for the credentialing and privileging activities of the medical staff, and the medical staff quality committee handles peer review. Some smaller medical staffs may opt to keep this work with the MEC, while larger medical staffs usually require different committees to carry out these functions.

Although these committees are the norm, regulatory/accreditation bodies do not mandate them.

In addition to committees, the MEC relies on the various department chairs to carry out medical staff activities. Department chairs are typically accountable to and report to the credentials and peer review committees. Many medical staffs also appoint the department chair to the MEC. The department chair makes recommendations to the credentials committee regarding an individual physician's medical staff membership and privileges. After review of the chair's recommendation, the credentials committee conducts its own assessment and makes a recommendation to the MEC. The MEC then makes a recommendation to the board.

THE MEC'S ROLE IN CREDENTIALING AND PRIVILEGING

The quality committee's work follows a similar path. An individual department chair is responsible for oversight of the quality of care provided by physicians in his or her department, but a centralized medical staff quality committee typically oversees peer review activity and is accountable to the MEC. See Figure 3.1 to better understand how the department chair and the committees relate to one another.

Before we delve into the MEC's specific role in the credentialing and privileging process, it's important to review the definitions of credentialing and privileging, because many people confuse the two topics.

What Is Credentialing?

Credentialing is essentially the verification of an individual practitioner's credentials—training and experience—to practice medicine. The credentialing professional verifies information regarding the practitioner's license, graduation from medical school, completion of an accredited residency training program, completion of fellowship training, board certification, malpractice insurance and malpractice history, and previous experience. Whenever possible, the information is primary-source verified through the organization that issued the document (diploma, certification, etc.). The credentialing professional can also turn to organizations that have been deemed the equivalent of a primary source, such as the AMA Physician Masterfile, to verify some information.

Credentialing may at first appear to be a fairly simple task, but a lot of careful work has to be done to ensure integrity of the information collected through the verification process. There are unscrupulous people out there who masquerade as physicians and physicians who are trained but may misrepresent themselves. The credentialing process aims to sniff these folks out and ensure that your organization does not allow them access to your patients.

What Is Privileging?

After the organization verifies a practitioner's credentials through the credentialing process, the next step is privileging that practitioner. Privileging aims to determine what a practitioner is competent to do within the institution. Data gathered through the privileging process allows the organization to match the privileges it grants to the physician with his or her current competence.

Demonstrated current competence is the single most challenging aspect of credentialing and privileging today. The bar has been raised from accepting that a physician was competent just because he or she failed to demonstrate incompetence. No longer is the philosophy, "No news is good news." In fact, The Joint Commission now requires hospitals to collect evidence of demonstrated current competence to ensure that privileging is an objective, evidence-based process.

THE MEC'S ROLE IN CREDENTIALING AND PRIVILEGING

All organizations, whether beholden to Joint Commission standards or not, should aim to collect evidence of physician competence to ensure that the organization provides exceptional patient care. Regulatory compliance is simply a byproduct.

Four Steps in the Credentialing and Privileging Process

Although complex, the credentialing and privileging process can be broken down into a four-step process.

Step 1: Establish policies and rules. In this step, the MEC must work with department chairs and credentials committee (ultimately approved by the governing board) to determine what constitutes the criteria for membership and the criteria for privileges, what constitutes a completed application, what references should look like, the process for delineating privileges, who evaluates and makes recommendations, and who has what authority. All these details must be determined when creating policies, rules, and procedures.

Step 2: Collect and summarize information. collect information and summarize it in what will ultimately be the completed application. This is primarily the responsibility of management. Credentialing professionals within the medical staff services department will take an application after a physician completes it, do the primary-source verification, query the National Practitioner Data

Bank, and collect malpractice carrier information and malpractice history. The medical staff services professional (MSP) also gathers references and identifies those references the department chair should make time to contact. The result of the MSP's initial work is a complete and verified application.

Step 3: Evaluate and recommend. We now have a completed application, and the department chair, credentials committee, MEC, and board must evaluate it to determine whether the applicant will be appointed to the medical staff and, if so, to which medical staff category and with what privileges.

The evaluation and recommendation process begins with the department chair. He or she reviews the application—the application could be for an initial appointment, reappointment, or new privileges or new technology for someone who is in between reappointment cycles. The chair's job is to evaluate the application using all of his or her clinical expertise. The department chair makes a recommendation regarding membership and privileges to the credentials committee. The credentials committee then makes a recommendation to the MEC. The MEC considers the recommendation and conducts its own review of he credentials files before making a recommendation to the board.

THE MEC'S ROLE IN CREDENTIALING AND PRIVILEGING

When evaluating a credentials file, don't rely solely on the MSP and department chair's review. Look for red flags, such as:

- Gaps in training or practice

- Previous corrective action

- Professional competence or conduct issues

- Incomplete or inaccurate information provided on the application

- Unusual requests based upon background or training

- Unusual background or training

- Multiple changes in practice sites

A red flag should go up if there are unexplained gaps, an unusually large number of malpractice cases, or a reference who opts not to answer a question. These issues may not signal a competency issue but should be investigated to be certain. Research why the practitioner has numerous malpractice cases filed against him or her, pull medical records when necessary, and ask questions about professional action taken against the practitioner by another hospital. You are entitled to ask for that additional information and should put the burden on the applicant to provide this detail.

When evaluating the credentials files, don't look only at gaps that might be fairly obvious, but also look at references. How do you evaluate references? There are often hints within the references that signal a potential issue. For example, the reference leaves something blank or rates all categories as excellent except for one. Read between the lines.

Risk stratify the application using the following scale:

- R-1: Clean applicants without "red flags"

- R-2: Applicants with minor issues that do not require ongoing monitoring

- R-3: Applicants with significant issues that require ongoing monitoring

Is there a minor bump that you've drilled down into and resolved? That's an R-2. Is this an application with a large bump or multiple bumps that everyone should note and to drill down into because it's not quite clear what those bumps mean? That's an R-3. Document the basis for your recommendations for all R-2 and R-3 applications and spend your time drilling down into these applications.

Step 4: Grant or deny. This includes deciding whether to grant or deny some or all of the physician applicant's requests. This final decision lies with the governing board. The board has the sole authority to grant medical staff membership and privileges. The

THE MEC'S ROLE IN CREDENTIALING AND PRIVILEGING

board also provides oversight of the medical staff's credentialing processes. Because the board is not typically comprised of healthcare experts/practitioners, members of the board rely on the MEC's recommendation regarding membership category and privileges for each individual applicant. As stated previously, the department chair makes his or her recommendation to the credentials committee, who issues a recommendation to the MEC. Privilege criterion recommendations follow a similar path.

Policy in Action

The credentialing and privileging process can be a bumpy road. To navigate the process, it is essential to develop and follow sound policies. An important tenet to keep in mind when wrestling with credentialing and privileging questions is, "Our policy is to follow our policy. In the absence of a policy, our policy is to create a policy." This "motto" is known as the "Five Ps." At first blush, it is a statement only a bureaucrat could love, but it does provide sound advice. Let's take it apart:

Our policy is to follow our policy.

This means that the organization commits not to do things on an *ad hoc* basis but instead consistently follow standard operating procedures.

In the absence of a policy, our policy is to create a policy.

What if we don't have a policy? What if the physician is requesting a privilege the organization has never before granted? The Five Ps tells us stop the process, take time to research the issue, design a policy, and then go back to evaluate the credentialing or privileging question that caused the committee to halt its work.

Essential Credentialing and Privileging Policies

Some of the policies the organization must adopt include:

- Creating privileging criteria

- Addressing new technology

- Resolving privileging disputes

- Evaluating low- and no-volume providers

- Expediting "clean" applications

- Addressing the use of telemedicine providers

- Assessing temporary privileges

Creating those policies is, as we said before, a step-one activity and needs to be done well. The MEC ultimately owns oversight responsibility for ensuring the adoption on sound credentialing and privileging policies and for ensuring that polices are consistently followed.

THE MEC'S ROLE IN CREDENTIALING AND PRIVILEGING

The MEC's job is to credential and privilege practitioners using all data available to predict his or her performance in the organization. It is impossible to make such a prediction with 100% accuracy 100% of the time, but good policies, good procedures, good data, and good leaders who evaluate the information arm the organization with critical tools. Remember, the governing board will almost always agree with the MEC's recommendations. The board depends on the MEC to do the right thing for the patients, the hospital, and the community.

CHAPTER 4

The MEC's Role in Peer Review, Quality, and Patient Safety

Although some physicians may assert that quality can't be measured, it has become increasingly clear over the past several years that healthcare organizations and providers must be accountable for the quality of care delivered. The MEC plays a critical role in defining, measuring, and improving quality and in turn holding individuals and the organization accountable.

The focus on quality increased in response to the rising cost of healthcare. People want to know what they are paying for when they receive medical care. They want to understand the connection between quality of care and cost of care. From a practical standpoint, the organization wants to provide the highest quality care possible at the most reasonable cost possible. The goal of quality improvement is to provide better quality at a lower cost.

To begin to tackle this challenge, the MEC first must understand a few basic definitions.

Quality: In essence, quality is compliance with standards. The MEC must agree on quality and patient safety standards and then determine to what extent the medical staff and the organization are complying with those standards.

Quality management: Quality management is process improvement—methods for improving performance and processes.

Patient safety: Patient safety is about minimizing errors and their impact on patients. That's the challenge. Humans make errors. Healthcare includes complex systems that are not always going to perform well. Addressing these inherent challenges is what patient safety is all about.

Utilization management: Utilization management is about making sure care is provided in the most cost-effective way possible.

Assigning Roles and Responsibilities

Consider the organizational chart discussed in Chapter 1. As you'll recall, the governing board provides oversight and delegates some responsibilities to the CEO, some to management, and some to the medical staff. The board primarily assigns to management the performance of systems and processes of care, and the board assigns the medical staff the quality of care that primarily depends upon the performance of individuals granted privileges. Therefore, the

THE MEC'S ROLE IN PEER REVIEW, QUALITY, AND PATIENT SAFETY

medical staff owns individual practitioner performance, with the MEC providing oversight.

The MEC's sphere of control is the quality of care delivered by members of the medical staff. Processes, systems, and patient safety efforts fall within the MEC's sphere of influence. To manage quality of care, the MEC must first define what it means to be a "good" physician within the organization. In other words, the MEC must set, communicate, and achieve buy-in to performance expectations. Consider the performance frameworks outlined in Figure 4.1 when developing these performance expectations:

Figure 4.1   **WHAT IS PRACTITIONER PERFORMANCE?**

Technical	Patient care
Service	Medical/clinical knowledge
Patient safety/rights	Practice-based learning & improvement
Utilization	Interpersonal & communication skills
Peer & coworker relations	Professionalism
Citizenship	Systems-based practice

The challenge for MECs is determining how to help the medical staff perform well in each of the dimensions of performance included in the above-described frameworks. To support the medical staff in achieving these performance goals, the MEC must ensure the right structures, processes, and policies are in place and commit to following the Power of the Pyramid described in

Chapter 2 (refer back to Figure 2.2). Remember, the Power of the Pyramid is a tool that allows the self-governed medical staff to hold peers accountable. In short, the first layer of the pyramid requires solid credentialing, privileging, and recruitment strategies. The following escalating layers of the pyramid are to set, communicate, and achieve buy-in to performance expectations; measure performance and provide feedback; manage poor performance; and lastly, if other steps fail to result in improved performance, provide corrective action.

The MEC's job is to make sure every layer of this pyramid is done well. However, the MEC does not carry out each layer of the pyramid but rather provides oversight of each step. Specifically, the MEC must:

- Develop and implement sound credentialing and privileging processes and look for opportunities to improve these processes

- Set performance expectations

- Ensure effective processes for measuring physician performance

- Review physician feedback reports and identify opportunities to improve these reports

- Develop and periodically assess the organization's process for managing poor physician performance

THE MEC'S ROLE IN PEER REVIEW, QUALITY, AND PATIENT SAFETY

- Gauge the medical staff organization's efforts to support physicians in their efforts to improve individual performance

- Ensure corrective action is taken only when necessary

Oversight of Ongoing and Focused Professional Practice Evaluations

There are several tools available to the MEC to assist in the monitoring of physician performance. The first is ongoing professional practice evaluation (OPPE). The Joint Commission introduced standards requiring OPPE several years ago and, although some organizations continue to iron out the kinks in their OPPE processes, we've begun to see the value in the data collected and monitored by this process.

In short, OPPE involves the continuous monitoring of physician performance to identify opportunities for improvement. To conduct OPPE successfully, the medical staff and quality departments must work together to collect and share data. When data indicate variation from expected performance, those data are looked at more closely through a process called focused professional practice evaluation (FPPE). For example, a physician's readmission rate may be higher than the accepted target number adopted by the medical staff. In such a case, the data may go to the peer review committee to conduct FPPE to determine the reason for the variation.

FPPE is also used for current medical staff members with new privileges or for those who are using new technology. FPPE is also used when someone is new to the medical staff. Remember, the term FPPE applies to several scenarios—when a potential performance concern is identified through OPPE and when the organization needs data to determine whether a practitioner is competent to carry out new privileges.

Managing Loose vs. Managing Tight

The job of the MEC is to balance physician success, hospital success, and good-quality patient care. To balance these goals, the MEC must strike a balance between managing loose and managing tight.

Managing loose is typically tied to allowing creativity, physician entrepreneurialism, and customized patient care to the patient. This management style also tends to lead to high levels of physician satisfaction. However, managing too loose, focusing too much effort on being "physician friendly," could negatively affect hospital success and patient care.

On the other hand, managing tight's value is standardization, high reliability, and cost-effectiveness. But a MEC that manages too tightly may make physicians slaves to the standards and inadvertently impede physicians' ability to earn a living or provide good care. Balancing these two management styles is an ongoing process that must be adjusted to tackle the challenges of the day.

Keep in mind that all organizations, not just medical staffs or hospitals, exist somewhere on the spectrum between the "manage loose" pole and the "manage tight" pole. Historically, healthcare's policy has been to manage loose, which resulted in too much variation and not enough standardization. As a result, healthcare has recently moved toward managing tight, with an increased focus on core measures, transparency, patient safety, and high reliability.

Further, medical staffs have long leaned to the "manage loose" approach and tolerated wide variations in clinical outcomes, cost-effectiveness, physician conduct, and noncompliance with policies. In other words, it would take a lot of work for a physician performance issue to rise to the top of the performance pyramid and result in corrective action. However, quality-of-care issues that were once tolerated will not be tolerated going forward. Accreditors, regulators, and patients are motivating this change toward a more "manage tight" approach. As a result, the MEC's role in overseeing physician performance through the peer review process, measuring performance, and providing feedback is increasingly important.

Managing Systems Performance

In addition to overseeing individual physician performance, the MEC must ensure systems and processes are operating effectively.

The quality of the organization's processes and systems has a direct impact on patient care. In fact, William Edwards Deming, who is considered by many to be the grandfather of the quality movement and continuous performance improvement fields, asserted that the vast majority of organizational quality issues were related systems and management—not individual performance.

There are three types of systems in most organizations:

1. **Operational systems:** How the organization gets work done

2. **Training systems:** How the organization prepares individuals to take their place in those operational systems

3. **Accountability systems:** How the organization sets, communicates, and achieves buy-in to performance expectations and then holds individuals accountable to those measures

Management of these systems is not in the hands of the MEC. The MEC owns only individual physician performance. However, the performance of each individual on the medical staff has a disproportionate impact on patient care. A physician's error or failure to follow a policy most likely has a larger direct impact on patient care than that of anyone else in the organization. Therefore, while individual physician performance is important, improving the systems in which the physician carries out his or her work is important. Systems improvement is within the medical staff and MEC's sphere of influence. The MEC must ensure that the medical staff is playing an appropriate role in improving systems.

Performance improvement models

MEC members must have a basic understanding of performance improvement models. There are various models implemented in healthcare organizations across the country—Six Sigma, Lean, PDCA. These are all models aimed at organizing the hospital's quality/performance improvement efforts. While we won't delve into the details of each of these models in this training, we will discuss the valuable shared elements of each of the approaches. Specifically, each model creates an organized structure around performance improvement. They establish a consistent method that brings together various players within the organization to work collaboratively to improve quality.

Further, these models stress that to achieve real performance improvement, the organization must commit constant attention to these initiatives. Performance improvement must be done in ongoing cycles. The organization identifies an improvement opportunity, assesses the issue, and develops and implements solutions. The issue is then reassessed to determine whether further improvements are needed. If so, the organization goes through the cycle again.

Successful performance improvement models also focus on creating a culture of measurement and stress the importance of measuring quality. The challenge for the MEC is sending the message to the medical staff that quality measurement and performance improvement is not about perfection. It is about continuously improving performance. Regardless of the level of the performance today, the organization expects that performance level—for the individual physician, the specialty, the hospital overall—to be higher a year from today. Again, it is important to send the message to the medical staff that the organization does not expect perfection in individuals or in the processes in which they work. No practitioner is perfect and no hospital is perfect. All organizations can do is constantly look for opportunities to improve.

Patient Safety Basics

The fact of the matter is that everyone—including physicians—makes errors. Some of these errors, like leaving your keys in the car, are minor. For physicians, a simple slip or lapse can potentially have a direct impact on patient care. That's why it's important that the organization develops barriers designed to catch such lapses. Consider the "Swiss cheese model" depicted in Figure 4.2. This model, based on a strategy described by James T. Reason in his book *Managing the Risks of Organizational Accidents*, illustrates several goals that will help the organization begin to develop a patient safety strategy:

- Reduce the number of holes/errors

- Strengthen the effectiveness of barriers to keep errors from impacting the patient

THE MEC'S ROLE IN PEER REVIEW, QUALITY, AND PATIENT SAFETY

Figure 4.2   **WHY DO EVENTS HAPPEN?**

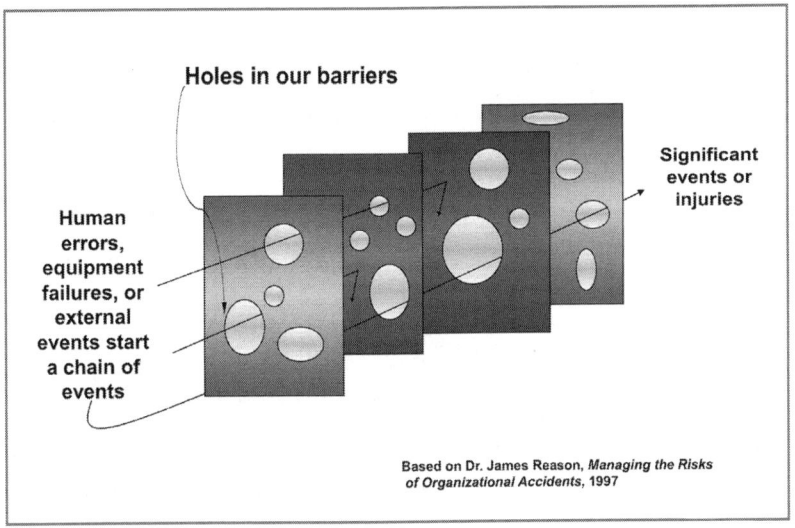

A slip or a lapse that occurs at the beginning of the process may occur simply because the practitioner did not follow a rule or process. The organization should have barriers in the place that detect the oversight or misstep from progressing. For example, barriers such as a checklist incorporated into the preoperate evaluation, a time out prior to the surgery start, or a pharmacist's review of a medication prior to dispensing. Just as no individual or process is perfect, no single barrier is perfect. That is why the organization should layer barriers to provide several opportunities to catch an error before it reaches the patient. Unfortunately, despite the best efforts, there are occasions when the holes in the Swiss cheese line up and an error adversely impacts patient care.

Four Components of Patient Safety

There are essentially four components that drive patient safety. The first components address changing processes.

Reactive improvements: The organization experiences a near miss, a sentinel event, or a series of events. As a result, it wants to investigate to determine why the near miss or event(s) occurred. This investigation is a root-cause analysis. The root causes of a near miss are often the same as the root causes of a sentinel event. Therefore, if an organization reacts to a near miss or a series of minor events and identifies the root cause and implements improvement processes, it can lead to proactive improvements to patient safety.

Proactive improvements: The organization does not have to wait for an adverse result, a near miss, or a sentinel event to happen to motivate patient safety improvement initiatives. Instead the organization looks at its processes to identify and then engineer opportunities for error. This is the approach taken by high-reliability organizations, and it is what a failure mode and effects analysis are all about.

The third and fourth components address changing behavior and the medical staff culture.

Behavioral expectations: The organization must set and communicate behavior expectations and accountabilities. As discussed previously in this handbook, medical staffs have long tolerated too much variation and lack of accountability.

Error reduction tools: Many organizations have adopted situation background assessment recommendation and other tools to reduce errors. In addition to these tools, the medical staff must support peer-to-peer coaching to hold each other accountable. For example, a physician would stop a colleague who entered an operating room in street clothes, but would that physician stop a colleague who did not wash his or her hands? Unfortunately, the answer to this question is too often "no." Coworker coaching is essential to achieving a culture of safety.

Implementing these four components reduces errors, results in high reliability, and improves safety.

Organizational Performance Improvement

Physician leaders can improve organizational performance by learning, understanding, and following the hospital's current improvement methods. Physician leaders can also drive quality improvement by defining goals and setting performance targets and then participating in organizational oversight of the performance improvement efforts. This oversight may take place at MEC meetings or hospital quality committee meetings. Either way, the physician representatives should be part of these discussions. The committees do not "own" performance improvement but rather oversee performance improvement initiatives.

Further, the MEC should participate in organized performance improvement teams when improvement opportunities are identified. Physician leaders should champion performance improvement activities and get buy-in from other physicians to ensure change and to secure physicians' commitment to hold themselves and others accountable for supporting that initiative.

It's important that the MEC understands the critical role physician leaders play in championing quality and patient safety, providing oversight of peer review, and participating in performance improvement. Hospitals with the best performance in patient safety and quality often have achieved that because physicians have not been dragged along reluctantly. Instead, physicians are taking the lead and making change happen.

CHAPTER 5

The MEC's Role in Managing Professional Conduct

Physician leaders have long struggled to effectively manage the professional conduct of their peers. A talented technically qualified physician who fails to conduct him- or herself professionally presents a sensitive, uncomfortable, and vexing challenge for MEC members. The first step in preparing to address unprofessional conduct is to understand the culture that allows such behavior to go largely unchecked.

The American Medical Association defines a problem physician as a physician who manifests behavior that directly interferes with or has a significant potential to undermine patient care and cause harm. The key point to take from that definition is the clear impact physician behavior has on patient care and the patient care environment. The MEC should not simply acknowledge that Dr. Smith "acts out" but must also acknowledge that Dr. Smith's behavior affects the care patients receive. The nursing staff may be uncomfortable communicating with Dr. Smith and therefore hesitate to alert the physician when patient care issues arise. The providers in the operating room may not communicate effectively as they focus on avoiding conflict with Dr. Smith rather than on delivering the best care. Whatever the case may be, the impact the physician's behavior has on patients must be documented.

Protecting a Culture of Safety

When examining physician behavior, the MEC must keep in mind that physicians have a duty and a right to alert the hospital of legitimate concerns regarding patient care, performance, skills, systems of care, staffing ratios, working conditions, or violations of legal and regulatory standards. The hospital must create a process that allows medical staff members to express concerns about the management team, nursing staff, and governing without fear of retaliation or punitive actions. Dissenting or pointing out opportunities for improvement is not disruptive or unprofessional behavior and must not be treated as such. The MEC must play its part in communicating that, in the organization's culture of safety, it is critical to create a culture of transparency and allow for an easy exchange of ideas free of fear of reprisal.

Legal and Regulatory Obligation to Address Conduct Issues

In 1991, Title 7 of the Civil Rights Act and Antidiscrimination Law first enacted in 1964 was expanded to include all organizations and

THE MEC'S ROLE IN MANAGING PROFESSIONAL CONDUCT

businesses with over 15 employees. The law states that treating an individual in a demeaning, disrespectful manner in the workplace may support a claim of discrimination under federal law, with compensatory and punitive damages.

The definition of a hostile working environment is drawn from this law. In short, any environment that undermines an individual's ability to do his or her job, including caring for patients, may constitute a hostile working environment.

Further, Joint Commission leadership standards introduced in 2009 require hospitals to create a culture of safety and quality that supports teamwork and respect for all members of the healthcare team. Keep in mind that teamwork and effective communication is central to building a culture of safety and quality. The only way for healthcare providers to communicate effectively and deliver quality care is through teamwork. It's one thing for a physician to write an order; it's another thing for all the members of the team to correctly carry out those orders and to communicate effectively with the physician and other healthcare practitioners when there is a change in clinical status. Therefore, physician behavior that intimidates and affects morale and turnover can lead to a breakdown in teamwork and harm patients. Medical staff leaders have an obligation to patients to intervene before that happens.

Create and Enforce Code of Conduct Policy

The organization should adopt a code of conduct policy that applies to everyone at the hospital—physicians, nurses, senior management, governing board, patients, and visitors. Everyone within the four walls of the hospital must be held accountable to maintaining a culture of safety regardless of their position in the organization.

The policy must define acceptable and inappropriate behavior and, most importantly, create a process for managing disruptive behavior. That process must detail the steps the organization will take at the first, second, and third instances of unacceptable behavior. The policy should set out time frames, expectations around performance, and consequences for failing to comply with the code of conduct policy.

As discussed earlier, the board delegates to the organized medical staff the responsibility to provide oversight and to improve the clinical quality and professional conduct of all practitioners granted privileges. The CEO oversees the system performance, which means if there is a professional conduct issue on the medical staff by either members or nonmembers privileged through the medical staff process, it is the MEC's responsibility to address. Although it is neither management's responsibility nor the responsibility of the chief medical officer, management can support the MEC in this endeavor. For example, the chief of staff may turn to the vice president of human resources for guidance and feedback on conducting an intervention.

Performance Pyramid to Address Conduct

The performance pyramid comes into play when the MEC addresses conduct. Credentialing and privileging is at the base of the pyramid. The best way to carry out these tasks is to adopt eligibility criteria for membership that include conduct, character, and ethics. Such criteria do not preclude the MEC from giving a practitioner with a history of disruptive conduct an application for membership and privileges. However, it does entitle the MEC to drill down and to find out the depth of the issue and its impact on patients and patient care. The same holds true at reappointment. Physician leaders can sit down with a physician who has exhibited unacceptable behavior, review the code of conduct policy with him or her, and ask that the physician sign the policy. If the physician refuses, emphasize that by filling out an application for reappointment, the physician has agreed to abide by all bylaws, rules, regulations, and policies, including the code of conduct policy. If the physician is unable to sign it or comply with the policy, he or she may be ineligible to reapply to the medical staff.

The next layer of the pyramid requires physician leaders to set, communicate, and achieve buy-in to expectations. At this step in the process, expectations about professional conduct should be articulated. For example, everyone in the organization must agree to treat one another with respect even at times of disagreement. Have practitioners who are struggling to meet this expectation sign the articulated expectation as a way to secure buy-in. And again, reinforce that federal law requires compliance.

The third layer of the pyramid is to measure performance against expectations. This step provides an opportunity to create a measurable indicator with targets around behavior and conduct. As part of measuring behavior, physician leaders must validate reports of unacceptable behavior. If a nurse reports a physician's unprofessional behavior, have a physician leader and a nursing leader sit down with both the physician and nurse involved as well as any witnesses to ascertain what happened and the impact, if any, upon patients.

You should have a behavioral indicator as part of your performance feedback report and as part of ongoing professional practice evaluation required by The Joint Commission. It's important that these measures are part of a physician's profile used to assess the physician's overall clinical performance and eligibility for reemployment.

As you near the top of the pyramid, the need to manage poor performance becomes more acute. The first step is collegial interaction, followed by a voluntary action plan, a mandatory action plan, and then a final warning. How quickly you implement a final warning depends on the egregiousness of the incident. Keep in mind that

THE MEC'S ROLE IN MANAGING PROFESSIONAL CONDUCT

some behaviors and actions require the organization to go straight to corrective action.

When the situation calls for corrective action, remember that if the organization takes corrective action that is less than 14 days, it is not obligated under the Healthcare Quality Improvement Act to provide that individual with due process rights (fair hearing and an appellate review by the board).

Although difficult, the MEC's role in managing physician performance is critical. The Joint Commission administered a sentinel alert that states that disruptive behaviors cause medical errors and deaths; increase costs, complications, liability, staff turnover, breakdown in communication; and are a leading cause of sentinel events. Also keep in mind that intervention is a means of offering support to a physician. Consider the wonderful general surgeon whose undiagnosed depression caused him to slam the phone down when a nurse contacted him in the middle of the night regarding a patient's condition. Because of the physician's standing on the medical staff, the nurse did not go up her chain of command and report the incident. On another evening, a patient with normal postoperative complications died because the nurse who was treated poorly in the past did not contact the physician to discuss the patient's deteriorating condition. The physician was then the subject of an intervention and consequently took a leave of absence and was treated for depression. When he returned to the medical staff, he turned to a physician leader who was a longtime colleague and asked, "Why didn't you help me all those years? I was struggling with depression." The chief of staff replied, "I thought we were helping you by looking the other way." This attitude is reflective of past medical staff culture. The MEC must now recognize that when it addresses behavior and conduct, it is helping physicians, patients, and the organization.

CHAPTER 6

The MEC's Role in Strategic Collaboration With the Hospital

The medical staff's strategic plan must detail how it will achieve an effective medical staff, help physicians succeed, help the hospital succeed, and provide great patient care. The MEC must guide the development of this strategic plan to allow the medical staff to effectively partner with the hospital to help it achieve its strategic plan. The two—the medical staff and the hospital—must work together to help one another succeed.

Unfortunately, not all medical staffs put forth the time and effort to create such a plan. But the fact is that the medical staff is one of the hospital's most important assets. The hospital has a plan to optimize the physical plant, human resources, and capital, but few have a formal plan to optimize the medical staff. However, a strategic medical staff development plan is a win-win for both the medical staff and the hospital.

A strategic medical staff development plan, in summary, can be referred to as "the seven Rs," which are the:

- Right number of physicians
- Right types of physicians
- Right quality
- Right relationship to the hospital
- Right medical staff culture
- Right structure and processes for the medical staff
- Right leadership

The seven "rights" help the hospital and the medical staff fulfill their mission and strategic plan. The MEC should be partnering with the hospital to help achieve just that. In the rest of this chapter, we'll walk through each of the seven Rs.

The Right Number

Establishing the right number requires a close look at the community the medical staff serves, the number of patients it serves, the demographics and ages of those patients, and the types of illnesses it treats. It also requires analysis of primary and secondary

THE MEC'S ROLE IN STRATEGIC COLLABORATION WITH THE HOSPITAL

service areas, out migration, and the medical staff roster. Further, physician-to-population ratios and physicians in the community that aren't on the medical staff must also be considered.

The Right Type of Physician

The element of the strategic plan is about individual specialties represented on the medical staff. To determine the right physician mix, the medical staff must look at specialty-to-population ratios, the primary care needs within the community, and the organization's plans to develop service lines. For example, the hospital may determine that it wants to grow its cardiovascular service line or create a women and children's health center of excellence. The hospital and medical staff must determine the right mix of physician specialties necessary to achieve those goals.

The Right Quality

The right quality depends on credentialing and privileging. The MEC must determine where to set the bar in regard to quality, credentialing, and peer review. The fact is that many organizations are dealing with the reality of the physician shortage. These organizations are put in the position of deciding whether to accept less-than-stellar physicians or accept that it won't have a particular specialty on its medical staff. Will the organization offer this service if it can't get a great physicians to provide the service? Will the organization compromise quality to serve the community or increase revenue? This is an important strategic discussion that must take place.

The Right Relationship to the Hospital

This is most often a specialty-by-specialty discussion that examines practice models and physician/hospital relationships. Are there a lot of private practice physicians in the community? Will the hospital employ physicians—young physicians seeking employment and/or older physicians that are struggling to keep their private practice successful? How will the hospital collaborate effectively with physicians if some are employed while others remain in private practice?

Contracts also come into play when determining the physician/hospital relationship. Contracts, such as exclusive contracts for radiology, pathology, and hospitalists, are increasingly common. Further, some hospitals are seeking out joint ventures, because such agreements ensure everyone has "skin in the game." Lastly, the medical staff must determine a strategy for low- and no-volume physicians, leadership development, recruitment, retention, and addressing competition. These are just a few of the issues the medical staff must examine when developing its strategic plan.

The Right Medical Staff Culture

Every medical staff culture has within it internal dynamics and tensions, including the following.

Collegiality and excellence. Collegiality is unconditional respect for each medical staff member. This respect abounds and is reciprocated among physicians. However, collegiality can sometimes impend improvement if physicians are unwilling to question the performance of others. This unwillingness may compromise excellence in such cases. However, the pyramid can help the organization achieve both collegiality and excellence.

Freedom and commitment. Physicians want to be free to make decisions regarding their practice and personal life, but they must be committed to the organization if they want a voice at the table and to expand their sphere of influence. They need to attend meetings, get and stay up to speed on issues, and participate in leadership activities.

Appropriate independence and mutual accountability. Mutual accountability is the essence of a self-governed medical staff. Physicians may push back on this idea and assert their independence to make clinical decision. Physicians are correct that they are highly trained and qualified to make independent decisions, which makes these tensions an ongoing challenge to balance.

Stability and change. Healthcare is changing at an unprecedented speed, and physicians must change with it. With all the change, we must take a step back and look at what medical staffs are doing well. Medical staffs can err on both sides of this equation. Some are afraid to change anything, while others are changing everything—including things that are working well. Further, a culture of continuous performance improvement (ongoing change) must acknowledge the medical staff's strengths and demonstrate appreciation for that work (stability).

The Right Structure and Processes

Organizations require effective bylaws, committees, departments, service lines, and physician councils. It needs thoughtful policies and procedures that guide the credentialing and privileging, peer review, and performance improvement processes. The MEC has the oversight responsibility to make sure the organization has this structure in place.

The Right Leadership

Leadership is essential in developing, implementing, and enforcing these policies. To foster strong leadership, the organization needs clear position descriptions, selection criteria, education and training, rewards and recognition, and succession planning. MEC owns oversight to make sure the organization is investing in physician leadership with all these elements in place. If they're not there, the MEC should be discussing them at their meetings and making them happen. Lastly, the MEC must openly discuss these tensions and help the organization balance them.

The Seven Rs are essential to creating an effective medical staff. It's the job of the MEC to provide oversight and ensure that all these aspects of an effective medical staff are in place. Management will do much of the detail work—from recruiting to number crunching—but the MEC owns the pieces related to medical staff culture, like structure, processes, communication, and leadership. The MEC must also find a way to collaborate with the hospital to achieve physician success, hospital success, and great patient care.

CHAPTER 7

Effective MEC Meetings

Understandably, busy physician leaders don't often take the time to learn the ins and outs of effective meeting management. However, this seemingly trivial issue can be essential to a leader's ability to get his or her job done. Poor meeting management skills result in 95% of medical staff meeting discussion focused on routine business rather than on important and challenging issues.

Developing the MEC Agenda

The first step in elevating the level of discussion that takes place at the MEC meeting is to create a consent agenda. Reports, issues, and announcements that don't require direct discussion and debate should go on a consent agenda. Any MEC member can request an item be moved from the consent agenda to the regular agenda for discussion. The first action taken at the MEC meeting is approval of the consent agenda. This simple move takes most routine business off the agenda and allows the meeting discussion to focus on the following.

Credentials committee recommendations on unusual and/or problematic applications. The credentials committee can also have a consent agenda for clean applications, and the MEC can put these clean applications through an expedited review and approval process. Don't focus the MEC's scarce time on routine credentials applications.

Unresolved or significant physician performance issues. When a significant performance issue comes before the MEC, allocate specific time frames to discussion of that issue. If the issue is not resolved or a game plan has not been agreed upon when the allotted time is over, it is unlikely that continuing the discussion will lead to a decision. Put the issue on the docket for the next meeting.

Concerns physicians want to communicate to administration. When the MEC wants to present concerns to administration, the group should discuss the issues at the MEC meeting with the goal of putting concerns in writing. Don't simply chat.

Reports from administration on the hospital's status and direction. Discuss only strategic reports that require discussion and debate. If it's a routine announcement from the CEO to the medical staff, put it on the consent agenda rather than assigning discussion time to the announcement.

Follow-up for implementation of the hospital strategic plan. The medical staff must be integrally involved in the hospital strategic plan, and there must be close communication between the MEC and the governing board. Therefore, the MEC may want to discuss strategic initiatives or strategic opportunities and challenges proposed by physicians or the hospital.

Many medical staffs have created physician councils out of frustration that the MEC meetings spend so much time dealing with routine business that there's no time to discuss critical, political, and economic issues affecting the medical staff. If the hospital does not have a physician council or if the MEC restructures it's meeting to allow more time for discussion of strategic issues, the group may spend meeting time addressing strategic questions, such as with whom to sign exclusive contracts, whether to build a surgical center, whether to align with an entrepreneurial physician group, whether to get into retail medicine, etc.

Reports from departments on key initiatives and challenges. Don't accept a department chair's assertion that he or she has nothing to report. There is most often something important going on in each department that should be shared with the MEC. The MEC must hold the department chairs accountable for their performance, so it is important that the MEC understands the chair's strengths, weaknesses, level of engagement, etc.

Assessment of the performance of contracted groups and outside services. This is a 2009 Joint Commission standard that states that the MEC has to be integrally involved in the content of contracts with all contracted services provided through the organized medical staff. Focus on strategic and critically important issues.

MEC Members' Role in Meeting Effectiveness

Once the agenda is developed, send it to MEC members one week before the scheduled meeting to allow for sufficient review of the agenda items. Although MEC members should review and understand the issues on the agenda when they arrive at the meeting, it is important to redistribute the agenda at the meeting.

Some MECs have adopted a strict policy that states that MEC members who come to the meeting unprepared to discuss the issues at hand are excluded from the discussion and final vote, the thought being that the vote should reflect the position of members who have read and carefully considered the agenda item.

In addition to arriving at the meeting on time, to aid meeting effectiveness MEC members should:

- Reach out to stakeholders prior to the meeting so to avoid "railroading" colleagues by passing an issue or initiative that will have a profound impact upon others before getting their input and achieving buy-in.

- Comply with conflicts of interest and confidentiality policies. Consider the chief of staff who is also the director of the emergency department. When a confidential issue arises at the MEC meeting that affects the emergency department, the chief should disclose his or her conflict to the group. The MEC members may ask the chair to share his or her input/insight into the issue but then step out of the room while the group has a confidential discussion and takes the vote.

- Speak up, but avoid dominating the discussion. It is important to hear from everybody, respectfully listen, and be willing to change your opinion. The main reason for having a meeting is to gather opinions to make decisions greater than the sum of the parts. The goal of MEC members is not to advance a personal agenda or sideline colleagues. It is to govern in good faith, maintain transparency, and usher in positive change.

- Come to the meeting with proposed solutions. For example, don't assert, "Nursing is bad." If there are opportunities for improvement, work with nursing leadership to come up with constructive initiatives to help improve nursing and the relationship between the medical staff and nursing. In other words, be part of the solution, not part of the problem.

- Commit time to work on MEC issues outside of the meeting. Remember, being a medical staff leader isn't just about attending meetings. It's about how physician leaders follow up, follow through, and take what is learned at the meetings to make a better medical staff.